POWER OF THE MIND

AND

PARKINSON'S DISEASE

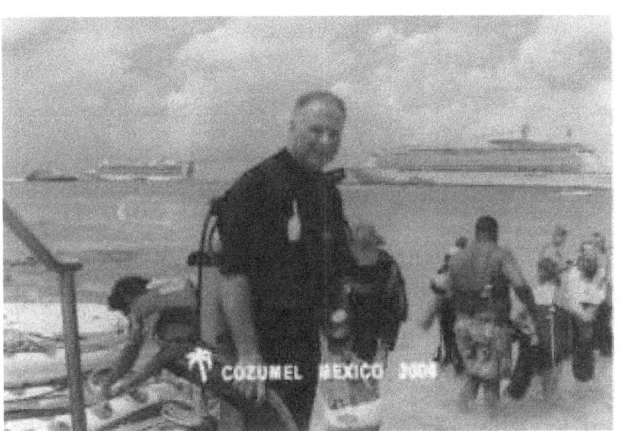

## Has your martial arts background been helpful once you were diagnosed?

*GORD SUMMER: Keeping fit was always important to me. In 1991 I started my spare time courier martial arts and today enjoy being a certified instructor and a 4.3 degree credential as a black belt martial artist. I am currently working to earn a full 4.4 credential by November 2011.*

© *Parkinsons Recovery*

# Power of the Mind

*Little did I know that the in-depth knowledge that I had acquired from my martial arts practice and training in Aiki Jujitsu would provide an unimagined, unique and powerful tool which has helped me harness the symptoms of Parkinson's.*

What is the most important tool that is needed to harness the symptoms of Parkinson's disease?

*GORD SUMMER: I believe it is the very simple word called calmness. When one is first diagnosed there is usually disbelief, fear and shock. Your mind is in a tailspin. You are overwhelmed with feeling sorry for yourself. Once you allow yourself to grieve the diagnosis, acceptance comes shortly after. Once you manage to go through this phase, the door opens up and Parkinson's becomes a "lease on life." My strong character allowed me to challenge this disease and move forward to extend my lease on life.*

# Power of the Mind

*Balance and calmness are important qualities that can be used to help you manage Parkinson's symptoms. Should achieving calmness not come naturally for you, I recommend that you train your brain and your nervous system to stay calm. Calmness lets you control deficiencies and harness them more easily. The "Power of the Mind" can harness your ability to be calm and balanced.*
*Calmness is, again, very important and it is extremely recommended that you truly search for calmness if it isn't natural for you.*

*Fifty percent (50%) of the "Power of the Mind" capacity is diminished when you are nervous. Calmness lets you control whatever deficiencies there are and harness them more easily. Our choice is simple. Allow this disease to overtake and shorten our lease on life or learn to achieve calmness.*

# Power of the Mind

**Do you tell strangers you have Parkinson's?**

*GORD SUMMER: For 13 years we worked with a Small Engines dealer who looked after our commercial lawn and snow removal equipment. One day in 2003 I walked into the dealership to have a chainsaw serviced. While sharpening the chains Aaron, the senior owner, took me aside and asked me. "Do you have Parkinson by any chance?" I confirmed! Aaron (a Mennonite through and through ) raised his voice and scolded me for not telling him. He told me that his son (age 40 then) had said to him: "The fire is out of Gord's eyes". They both wondered if I was in financial trouble, if my marriage had dissolved or if I was sick. Ever since then I freely divulge my condition.*

*I would like to share with you how I handle this potentially embarrassing situation. Many people with Parkinson's experience a staring problem. Instead of waiting for an uncomfortable reaction, I*

© Parkinsons Recovery                    4

*like to dispel that uneasiness and take the guesswork out of a person's thoughts by simply saying - particularly to the ladies - that "I am awkward, stiff and I do stare. I apologize for that. It is a medical condition called Parkinson's. Please, kindly ignore."*

*The reason for divulging that information is to keep everyone, including myself, comfortable should symptoms such as staring create a concern for anyone. Parkinson's is not something easily hid. Putting people at ease before any misunderstandings achieves calmness.*

*This gesture puts me at ease and helps me become calm. Simply put - I am telling them this is me. I can live with it. Can you? I am able to put the saved energy to better use by controlling symptoms with the "Power of the Mind".*

*In a visualization that was very revealing I realized that I was feeling sorry for myself - short of being depressed. I was letting*

# Power of the Mind

*Parkinson's have its way with me. Simply put, I was allowing Parkinson to win over me.*

*I said to myself "no way." Defiant - I turned 180 degrees and kicked myself literally in my own behind with the words, so what? I am still alive. I have 30 years still to go. Many people cross the streets and never make it to the other side. People around me who were 45 to 60 years old were dropping dead. I realized that in reality, I had a lease on live. I set the intention to make the utmost of it. Even better than that, the thought was born to fight Parkinson and win, to get rid of it!*

*I teach Ju Jitsu and am experienced in the various martial arts like Judo, Karate and Tai Chi. JuJitsu by the way means gentle heart. After doing 108 moves of Tai Chi every evening I would use a grounding procedure with my eyes closed as an opportunity to appeal to my sub conscious to get healthy, substitute dopamine with other ways to move and even better, get rid of Parkinson's . After a few months it became clear to me that I had gained knowledge in the last 12 years on my way to a 3rd degree black belt and certified instructor that I could utilize to control and win over Parkinson's.*

How have you used the "Power of the Mind" to reverse your symptoms?

*GORD SUMMER: Yes. I have been using various methods that were borrowed from my martial arts training to channel energy from strong parts of my body to the points of short fall. While doing so it crystallized in my mind that the moving of a resistant left arm with its adjoining hand and fingers or getting my left leg to walk was related back to the use of the "Power of the Mind". From here on I began to utilize and access the "Power of the Mind" on demand to facilitate movement of my body.*

*This ability came to its real test in 2008*

*during my Rescue Diver test while I was under water. I wanted to become a certified Rescue Diver very badly. The test was a genuine challenge. I began to run out of dopamine during the final two minutes of the underwater test. I appealed to the "Power of the Mind" to move regardless of the deficiency. I was very desperate and wanted to succeed for personal as well as family reasons. I am a fighter who never gives up. I gave it everything I had, including substituting the missing dopamine with adrenaline as well as borrowing energy from other body parts using the "Power of the Mind" martial arts style. I passed the test. The underlying message is : Never give up ! THE ONLY ONE THAT CAN STOP YOU IS YOURSELF !*

## How do you access the "Power of the Mind"?

*GORD SUMMER: [Short Version]: To illustrate the "Power of the Mind" we can turn our attention to the experience we have all had sitting in the most dreaded dentist's chair. The anticipation of awaiting a tooth to be drilled without sedation creates much anxiety and fearful thoughts. Using the "Power of the Mind" to calm and train your thoughts can release endorphins within minutes to sedate your tooth and keep you from jumping out of your chair from pain.*

*[Long Version]: Think about occasions when you have been sitting in a dental chair waiting to have a tooth drilled. You decide not to have Novocaine so the drilling is without sedation. The drill comes closer and closer to the live nerve. Pain increases along with your anxiety. Your thoughts go towards "I wish the pain would go away."*

*Suddenly, you become calmer. The pain is reduced and becomes more tolerable. "Power of the Mind" sends in the endorphins. Once you have trained your mind to access the "Power of the Mind" on demand you can sedate your tooth within minutes.*

*This is the very same "Power of the Mind" that can be used to channel Ki energywithin your body. "Power of the Mind" can be used as an important, effective weapon against Parkinson's.*

*When you work with Ki energy there are communications between cells that are electrical currents. Ki energy can be used to alter these electrical currents. The body is divided in two parts; a left and a right side. I take the Ki energy from the strong side of my body and shift it over to the weak side of my body.*

*I learned this energy technique in Aiki quite accidently when my arm did not want to co-operate as I was trying to get food from the plate to my mouth. I pointed my left pinky finger (the small finger on my left hand) away from my fork. Although this may sound strange, I then channeled the Ki energy from my brain through my arm into my hand and then into the pinky. My arm begins to take the food from the plate to my mouth.*

*Using this method at the table became second nature to my family at meal time. It took about two on months using that method to reinforce the realization for me that the "Power of the Mind" is a powerful tool which offers immediate results.*

*When you have Parkinson's, you get the sensation that one or the other arm has turned into a paperweight. My left arm can feel like a paper weight while my right arm remains fairly healthy and strong. I access the "Power of the Mind" to drive the Ki energy down the entire right side of my body. Then I channel this infusion of energy over to my left side. My mind literally goes down the left arm right into the finger tips. There is a slight tingling and the "Power of the Mind" energizes the left hand by automatically borrowing energy from the other extremities on the right side of the body. The left hand starts to execute the desired movement.*

*My left hand starts calming down. Tremors vanish. My voice starts to sound monotone, but that is a small price to pay. I look as if nothing is wrong with you. I am convinced that Ki energy does suppress symptoms.*

*To speed up the process I utilize controlled breathing by rolling my tongue back towards the throat. It sounds a little like throttled breathing. This increases and multiplies the energy to the left arm to achieve the desired result. Using this method repeatedly becomes second nature.*

*Simply turning the blinker lever of my car was sometimes problematic. The lever (which is on the left side of the steering wheel) became a challenge when my hand suddenly decided to freeze. My determination decides otherwise. I used Ki energy to solve this problem by taking a short inhale breath, placing my tongue on the back of my throat and exhaling with a quick, short breath that sounds like a loud power burst. When powering my hand with Ki energy using the breath, I am able to move the blinker any which way I wanted. If you try it, I'm certain you will find that it works.*

*Let me now explain how I use the "Power of the Mind" to help me walk without effort. Sometimes my left foot drags behind the right. I can feel the dopamine level is low which forces me to be conscious of walking properly. I first shift my weight from the upper body down towards my hip bone. Then I shift the lower pelvis forward, pull my shoulders back and make the adjustments needed so that my body is supported by the center of gravity. My steps get noticeably longer and faster. I am moving without much notice to others. Again, the "Power of the Mind" is at work.*

# Power of the Mind

*I have demonstrated this technique many times. Let's say you stand on both feet, tall and upright. I'm sure you learned as a child to be a potato bag which means that your mind tells your body to get heavy. If somebody wants to throw you off balance, your natural instinct is to get heavy. You get heavy, unlock you knees and bend a little bit forward. Then you shift your pelvis forward which may remind you of marital duties. This means you lower yourself a little bit in height. Then you start walking. Try it. You might be surprised at the result.*

*Remember, Parkinson's likes to lock out your trunk, which means some of your bones are not exactly in the place they are supposed to be. Stiff muscles always pull on the skeleton. Stand tall. Get heavy (which means you lower yourself a little bit). Sink down a little bit. Allow your knees to go a little bit forward. Shift your pelvis forward and then walk. You will find that you get quite a speed accomplished - so much so that your family will have difficulty keeping up with you all the time.*

*Whether through meditation or breathing techniques we can communicate with the subconscious.   When that feeling of running out of dopamine appears, I appeal to the mind to get me moving to complete my task.  It takes approximately two minutes. Ninety percent (90%) of the time I am able to carry on with the physical work I do.*

*I wish to strongly emphasize the worthwhile task of trying to find access to the "Power of the Mind".  You will be surprised how you can improve and manage and almost overlook the idea that you have Parkinson's.  I am serious and not being dismissive in questioning whether medication is necessary, often thinking "I'm feeling so good, why do I need it?" Yes, I encourage you to see how the "Power of the Mind" can be beneficial.*

# Power of the Mind

*You have probably all experienced accessing the "Power of the Mind" without realizing it. While driving a car you suddenly notice something is not right quite with your hands. After clapping your hands over the steering wheel very briefly two or three times you detect that your hands are obeying you. Without knowing it, you have tapped into the "Power of the Mind". A strong desire to access this will bring positive results. Rest assured that this method should assist you in moving forward and not looking back.*

Can a novice use "Power of the Mind" successfully?

*GORD SUMMER: Familiarity with the method makes it easy for me; however, a beginner can learn how to use the "Power of the Mind" by doing the meditations. Sit or stand calm with closed eyes. Do breathing techniques similar to yoga. You will find that your fingers start to prickle. You will feel a very fine tickling in your fingers. When you look at your hands you will see a marbling - white and red spots will appear throughout the palms. Appeal for calmness. Exercise these procedures. Suddenly, the "Power of the Mind" opens the door to greater calmness, enhanced mobility and greater flexibility.*

*I achieved wonderful results using martial arts principles of Aiki which activates the electrical current between cells using the techniques of breathing and tightening up the body. I can grab your hand by the wrist and send an electrical current to your body which will feel like a powerful jolt. The energy can be so powerful that some people are thrown up in the air and come crashing down on their back.*

*This may sound a little bit odd but once you manage to achieve opening the door to the "Power of the Mind", you will be stunned at what you see. It is extremely powerful. People use only ten percent of what can be available to us.*

# Power of the Mind

*An example of this strength was when a hospital endured a serious fire. Once the fire came close to the section with Parkinson's patients in residence, they hurriedly got up and ran across the street. Once safely across the street, they froze and fell down. An explanation for this remarkable feat is that the "Power of the Mind" ordered the body to substitute dopamine with adrenaline to get everyone moving.*

*Another example of how people automatically harness the "Power of the Mind" became evident I spoke with my Doctor in Seattle about the placebo effect in drug trials. The "Power of the Mind" is very evident in medical trials. To evaluate the effectiveness of new medications, some patients are given the Real McCoy while others are given a placebo. It is evident that within a few months all involved in certain trails seem to be improving, whether they are taking the real drug or placebo.*

# Power of the Mind

*What is really happening here is the desire to prevail, believing that you have something that will enhance your quality of life. You can sense improvement solely because you believe you will get better. The "Power of the Mind" is the actual medication.*

Have other members in your family been diagnosed with Parkinson's?

*GORD SUMMER: Since my father had Parkinson's I was very familiar with his symptoms and what he had gone through. Although I was not diagnosed until 2003 I became suspicious of my symptoms years earlier in July 1999. I noticed a very fine pain going through the left arm as I drove my car with my arm resting on the window sill. I knew that time would reveal itself. My hunch proved correct with a diagnosis of Parkinson's in 2003 since my father started out with these same symptoms. Although some believe that Parkinson's is not hereditary – I do have to smile since I believe it is very much in our genes. Somehow, mother nature decides to mess with those genes and make us receptive to certain conditions.*

**What has been your history of Parkinson's symptoms?**

*GORD SUMMER: How did I manage to function for four years - from 1999 to 2003 – before I was diagnosed the first time officially? It was called CoQ-10 or Coenzyme 10. Believe it or not, with 60 mg in the morning and 100 mg later in the day, my Parkinson's symptoms disappeared for almost four years. I managed my symptoms well using CoQ10, later increasing the dose to 200 mg.*

*Once I was diagnosed, I noticed that my left hand shook and the trunk of my body appeared stiff. When scuba diving in 2006, it felt as though I were a tree stump underwater. Parkinson's wrapped around my body, very slowly in my case, leaving my left foot dragging. While in Cuba, it took a very special person, my five year* old grandson, who walked with me a short distance at the resort. My grandson suddenly hit me with his hands behind my upper thighs on my left leg and he said, "Move, move, move!" I realized that I needed to listen to what a little five year old was teaching me.

In my quest for a second opinion I was fortunate to connect with Dr. Monique Giroux in Cleveland, Ohio. After the initial examination she looked me square in the eyes and said, "You know you have Parkinson's." She told of her experience in treating over 2,000 people a year. From the first dose of medication prescribed to me, I was impressed with her reaction. When I was concerned about how my left foot dragged a little bit she emphasized that it was necessary to "be reasonable now and prettier would come later."

I later gained a new trust in how true her words were. I must say that ten years later living with Parkinson's, my symptoms are better than when I was first diagnosed.   This serious journey meant learning many new lessons.

## What therapies proved to be useful?

GORD SUMMER: Parkinson's does not mean you isolate yourself, feel sorry and slowly fade away.  No, Parkinson's is a lease on life and your opportunity to stay very active, defiant and stubborn. Defiance was a strong quality that proved beneficial in fighting my symptoms. I found that sitting for long periods of time doing accounting work made me stiff. I would try to reduce the impact of this unfortunate reality by using Thai massage.

My visit to the Thailand Koh Tao diving center in 2008 to see whale sharks proved that my body was responding too slowly. Noticing how slow and stiff I was during the dive excursion, my teachers recommended a Thai massage.  I was aggressively handled by three people; one *on my feet, one on my arms and one on my back. After noticing my medical bracelet with the word Parkinson's, my treatment changed. I then needed to use the "Power of the Mind" to put myself into a half-asleep mode so I could withstand the pain of the pulling and stretching for an hour. Their concern was expressed to my wife who reassured them that I knew how to manipulate my body in order to withstand the pain of the rough treatment.*

*Soon after I got up off the floor, I put my undershirt on and shook my body like a young lad who automatically slid his shirt down. The warm, sticky climate did not hamper my instant surge of energy as I was greeted and admired with cheers and clapping by my therapists. Evidence of my flexibility reinforced the progress of their good work.*

*I am a firm believer in <u>Homeopathy</u>. Although my former family physician* *labeled them as a charlatan, I beg to differ. However, it is very important to me to keep a good relationship with my family doctor. I find that what modern medicines tend to destroy, the homeopathy pieces together. It seems that it goes full circle to the kidneys, heart, lungs and other organs. I am grateful that both modalities work well for me.*

*Tai Chi can also be beneficial. This produces balance and coordination between the mind and body. It is an authentic demonstration of the "Power of the Mind" over matter.*

*On a day when you're stiff and dragging your foot, the 108 moves which you can learn in three to five months is very helpful. If you are a serious beginner, you can start building and fine-tuning the 108 moves within 3 months and learn how to ground yourself. This is the best way to communicate with the "Power of the*

# Power of the Mind

Mind" if you're really serious about doing it on a daily basis. I am able to do the 108 moves in about 15 minutes whenever I go down to my space in the basement. Within five minutes on my worst day I am able to feel the effects of my extremities starting to conform. After ten minutes, you start to smile and everything is working for you. When completed after 15 minutes you walk like a puppy with energy and no ill effects. I would suggest it is worthwhile learning this.

It is extremely important that you develop a trusting relationship with your doctor. Search for a doctor who you can connect with. I am fortunate to have connected with a phenomenal lady, Doctor Monique Giroux. She takes plenty of time. It only takes 20 or 30 seconds to decide what I need but she still takes unrushed time to talk about what concerns me. It took me less than 10 minutes meeting this doctor to know and trust her for my life choices. I remember sharing my enthusiasm of my *martial arts to the Doctor and nurse as I stood like the Karate Kid with kicks that brought smiles to their faces.*

*Having a good night sleep is important. The moment I awake I have a goal in mind for the day. Generally, 5 or 6 hours gives me a proper rest but sometimes I often run on 5 hours a day.*

> **Is having Parkinson's symptoms a gift or a curse?**

*GORD SUMMER: When people first hear that I have Parkinson's the most common reaction is: "I am so sorry." I do not engage in sympathy. Parkinson's has gifted me with the ability to be patient and more understanding of others. I view it as a lease on life. Parkinson's and positive thinking has given me the ability to communicate with seniors at a different level. While we appreciate that the nursing home business is our family's bread and butter I have been able to see firsthand those experiencing similar* handicaps such as the ability to get the food from plate to mouth.

Since 2004 I was able to use a side line of martial arts, called Tai Chi and learned all 108 moves. Being a martial artist, I was able to absorb the details in no time which surprised the Taoist organization.

I enjoy entertaining my wife to show her that through the breathing techniques you can create energy and channel it from one extremity to another. I put my hand out, did the breathing, pushed her with her chair tilted and then slowly let her come back.

In the early days of looking fragile, many people were surprised that I could manage to harness my disability so well. Even more startling was walking up to them with my arm out against them and said, "Push." The Ki energy and breathing technique prevented them from pushing my arm to my body or pushing me at all.

# Power of the Mind

*There are no guarantees in life for anyone, with or without Parkinson's. Having a positive mind and staying active often results in forgetting to take your medication because your mind is distracted. It is exciting to realize that not taking a missed dose did not really make any difference.*

*As a martial artist, I always scan myself every couple of seconds. Often the message comes back that my '"good" arm is a paperweight. I refuse to accept this as a problem and command the "Power of the Mind" to "shut up and take notice." My best arm needs to be fixed and able to move.*

*My persistence pays off when I refuse to acknowledge that my arm cannot move. My arm is not a paperweight. In the worst of circumstances my weak arm is still 70% capable of what my strong arm is capable of doing. Before my diagnosis of Parkinson's both arms had equal strength.   On a good day, I have 80%, 85% almost 90% use of my weaker arm. Since 2011 my left arm is capable to perform over 90% what the right can. However, strength wise "the left arm" has surpassed the right arm.*

## What medications are you presently taking?

*GORD SUMMER: I smile to say that I take 6 mg per day of what I call "the gambling drug" Miraplex.  It has no negative effect on me.   There was the shopping urge. However, I soon determined with the "Power of the Mind" that I didn't need this nonsense.   It worked for me.*

*I also take Amantadine, 300 mg three times a day – seven o'clock, noon and 5 pm.  Since 2008 I have taken Sinemet 25 - 100 which is the combination of Cardopa and Levadopa .  I also take  one Stalevo - 200 / 100 / 25 [Entacapone / Levodopa / Carbidopa] since March of 2010  at 5PM only .*

# Power of the Mind

*Since 2008 I have taken the same medications without an increase or decrease in dosage with the exception of substituting Sinemet at 5 pm with Stalevo . I feel I should start to reduce.*

*On September 24, 2011 the first reduction occurred. I was able to eliminate the intake of Stalevo, returning to the former intake of Sinemet instead. It was clearly noticeable two weeks later that the desire of involuntary movements which I was suppressing by the use of the "Power of the Mind" started to fade away.*

**Tell us about your experience with the certification process for Master Diver**

*GORD SUMMER: I needed a certificate from the neurologist to scuba dive. The only concerns I faced in having Parkinson's and diving was the uncomfortableness of the instructors who were cautious about granting me a license. My stubbornness and insistence paid off as they threw me over the pier with all the gear on. Once in the water my feet did not want to cooperate with providing the proper propulsion. I was in the water for almost three hours with everything on - the weights, the BCD (buoyancy control device) but with no tank or breathing apparatus regulator.*

*The instructor looked over the wall and in amazement asked "Are you still alive? You must be exhausted by now." My message back to the instructor was the following. "Do what you have to do to prepare me." Impressed with my determination, they agreed to work with me as in Karate camp. I was soon awarded the open water license.*

*I was always invigorated after coming to the surface after a dive underwater after 30, 50 or 60 minutes (depending on the depth I was in). After getting back on land I marched around as if nothing was wrong for 20 minutes, feeling like a new born with my hands and feet working properly.*

© *Parkinsons Recovery* 31

# Power of the Mind

My certification is Master Diver which is a recreational certification. Dive Master and Instructor is a professional degree. Before you can get your Master Diver certification, you have to be certified as a Rescue Diver. To get this certification I had to complete a series of challenging tasks: going under water and rescuing people, bringing them up to the surface, towing them, giving them rescue breaths, undressing them, taking their equipment off and towing them ashore against currents. Yes, against currents.

During the test to be certified as a rescue diver in May 2008 I ran out of dopamine while underwater. The current was beginning to push me back. I ordered my left foot to move through the "Power of the Mind." I was so desperate to get the license that my mind helped my body substitute adrenaline for the dopamine deficiency. For two minutes I was riding on something other than dopamine, but my goal was met. I was certified as a *rescue diver.*

*I have also experienced the power of accessing Ki energy while swimming with a snorkel in my mouth in a swimming pool. I was lying without moving in the middle of the pool as if I were a statute. I had a three-quarter dive suit which helped me float well so I was not in danger. My left arm did not want to give me the courtesy to swim further. With the snorkel in my mouth I did the Ki energy deep breathing. While doing so, my arm obeyed me and I began to swim using the traditional swim stroke - forward, back and triangle. I came to the other side along the pool without little effort or strain.*

*When I explained my difficulty to the lifeguard, he reported that he had not noticed anything unusual. Again, using the "Power of the Mind" in conjunction with the Qi breathing technique allows you to succeed where others may give up.*

> **Does it help you to push your body to the point of exhaustion?**

*GORD SUMMER: Yes. I personally think it is a very good thing to do. I set a goal in my mind and I want to achieve it. The way I accomplished my goal was to increase my physical activities. For example, I used a pick and a shovel to dig a hole that was needed for a pipe project. I learned how to drive a bobcat and how to use a small swing shovel. I immersed myself in real construction work.*

*You start to get exhausted. Then you tap into your tenacity. After about five or six hours of working hard I would access the "Power of the Mind" to go beyond, pushing myself beyond my usual limits.*

*The easiest way to explain how I would push myself to the point of exhaustion is to describe how I would run around the block in my neighborhood. When I am out of shape it takes me 9 minutes 30 seconds to run the 1.4 kilometers (or .9 miles) around my block. Over the course of 14 days I would push myself to my limit. I would literally be gasping for air as I ran. I would continue pushing further and harder, regardless. After 14 days I could run around my block in 7 minutes 20 seconds.*

*I am always richly rewarded after pushing myself to the point of exhaustion. How? I walk the next day as if I were a young lad. Everything functions better. Blame it on better circulation. Blame it on the better blood flow through your system that is enriching parts of your body with more nutrients. Perhaps those explanations can best be left to a doctor.*

*Pushing yourself to the point of exhaustion certainly loosens your body. It makes stiffness take a backseat. It leaves Parkinson's easily behind for an entire day. This has certainly been my personal experience.*

*Let's assume you are a couch potato.*

# Power of the Mind

*Start running around the block or on a treadmill. Go as far and as long as you can. Then, let a few hours go by or the next day. If you do heavy workouts on treadmills or if you run, do it every other day to give your body a rest. Do some other activity or sport. Try to use different muscles than the day before. You will notice over time that when you do these strenuous tasks, your time will improve. Your heart will beat less vigorously and you will gain strength. Your steps will get longer and you will no longer shuffle along as you walk.*

*When I walk I also use the "Power of the Mind" to make myself heavy. I unlock my knees, shift my center of balance and push my pelvis forward. My steps then get longer.*

## Has CoQ-10 been helpful?

*GORD SUMMER: Coenzyme Q-10 has come a long way since the time when I first used it in the first three or four years* to stabilize Parkinson's and without doubt works.  I take a form called _Coenzyme Q-10 Ubiquinol_.  Ubiquinol is a form of Coenzyme Q-10 that is able to penetrate the blood brain barrier. It is fully absorbed by the brain. I take 1200 mg a day of a water soluble form of Coenzyme Q-10 Ubiquinol that I acquire from _Inno-vite_ (_http://www.inno-vite.com)._ I know it can calm down the symptoms of Parkinson's for several years.  I also have noticed there are negative days when I have not taken it.

Is there a connection between CCSVI and Parkinson's?

GORD SUMMER: _CCSVI_ [Chronic Cerebrospinal Venous Insufficiency] has actually made its way around the world just a year ago.  The term refers to compromised blood flow to the brain due to blockages in the jugular vein. **Error! Bookmark not defined.**These are the drain pipes that bring blood from the brain back to the lungs and then to the *heart. Lack of blood flow has been theorized to be a factor which can cause the symptoms of Multiple Sclerosis (MS).[1]*

*Why should compromised blood flow to the brain be a factor that might also cause symptoms of Parkinson's? I felt the connection was metal poisoning. Let me explain by way of an example.*

*When a river flows from the mountain tops, the water takes on significant rubble and sediments. Once the water reaches a valley the river slows down, so the water naturally drops impurities. The same happened in my left brain. The blood*

---

[1] *Chronic Cerebrospinal Venous Insufficiency (CCSVI) is a recent medical term developed by Italian researcher Paolo Zamboni in 2008 to describe compromised flow of blood in the veins draining the central nervous system. Zamboni hypothesized that CCSVI plays a role in causing the symptoms of multiple sclerosis (MS). Dr. Zamboni's wife was stricken with MS. He determined that both of her jugular veins were seriously compromised and thus theorized that her MS symptoms were due to an insufficient blood supply to her brain.*

*could not flow from my brain through my left jugular vein (the brain's drain pipe) because it was closed. My body thus had no way to cleanse heavy metal impurities that had been deposited in my brain.*

*My homeopathic doctor took hair samples in 2003 and 2005 which were sent to a lab in Chicago for analysis. I suspected than I had quite a nice gathering of heavy metals in my body. Results proved my suspicion to be correct. Significant deposits of arsenic, mercury and aluminum (to list only a few) were found. Even though my family doctor for 19 years until 2005 thought that this was a crock and that my homeopathic doctor was a charlatan, my intuition proved to be correct.*

*Heavy metals have been found to be present in people with Parkinsons, Alzheimer's, MS, people with allergies, incurable lung disease autism etc. etc. etc... Knowing that the tests had shown I had significant deposits of heavy metals, I drew a parallel between the compromised blood flow to the brain for MS patients and my own Parkinson's symptoms. .*

*An MRI – CCSVI under Doppler was performed over one and a half hours in Vancouver, British Columbia by AIM Imaging. The doctor looked at me after the MRI and said, "How the hell did you come to that idea to go the multiple sclerosis way as a Parkinsonian ?" I asked whether he had found anything. He just turned the screen around and showed me the results.*

*My left jugular vein was 9 mm shut. Also visible on the MRI were metal deposits surrounding the substantia nigra, disabling dopamine production and holding production hostage. I expected that my substantia nigra would have been very tiny. I was surprised to see that my substantia nigra was about 80% intact.*

*Shortly after the diagnosis a minor invasive surgery was performed by Pacific*

*Intervention in Los Angeles A by Dr. Todd Harris, who opened my jugular vein. The surgery involved entering the main vein in my groin area and feeding a balloon through the heart right into the jugular vein. Once in the correct position the balloon is popped. The artery opens the vein and flow to the brain is cleared.*

*While recovering I made motions with my fingers in front of the TV as if I was composer of a large music concert. My wife soon noticed my voice had gotten louder and the pace of my talking stepped up. Yes, my walking became brisker. Over the coming month the so much hated staring would slowly improve.*

*Now the task was to clear Heavy Metal Detox which I proceeded to do. Would I do it again? These questions are for you to ponder, however I personally would do it again, any day. Does it eliminate Parkinson's? I don't know. Does it reduce the symptoms? I feel it was very beneficial. It has made me feel like I was on top of the world.*

*I am thinking now I am in a position to begin reducing my medications.  I eliminated my 5 o'clock medication for three days without noticing any difference.  When I took the medication I started to slow down.*

## Have you found glutathione to be helpful?

*GORD SUMMER: Glutathione has a regulatory effect on the nervous system, brain function, oxygenation, detoxification and the immune function. It is often recommended as a treatment for the symptoms of Parkinson's. Dr. Monique Giroux pointed out that Glutathione is best administered with a nasal spray applicator. Oral glutathione is a waste of your money because it is processed by your digestive system before it can even reach the blood stream.*

*After a long search on the internet I found a source for glutathione nasal spray at*

*GlutaSource.com. I now use two products from Gluta Source: glutathione nasal spray and their suppository. I insert the 500 mg Suppository Formula before bed time, evenings only. I use the Glutathione nasal spray as needed.*

*Positive changes from taking Glutathione in the form of suppositories and nasal spray have been apparent from the first week of application. I had more energy. My Parkinson's symptoms were reduced. I was more alert behind the steering wheel. When the dopamine tank is low, I spray the Glutathione in each nostril and things look up for the better. I continue to improve month by month.*

**What would you say to a person who has just been diagnosed with Parkinson's?**

*You must believe that your life is worth living. You must not give up and withdraw from society and activities.*

**How to Hear Gord Summer on Parkinsons Recovery Radio**

Visit
http://www.blogtalkradio.com/parkinson
s-recovery *and scroll back to find the show
that aired December 29, 2010 featuring
Gord Summer as my guest.*

## About Gord Summer

*I began my life's journey in Europe as
a farmer's son 60 years go.  That
experience led me to acquire my
education as a master agriculturalist.
However, for 27 years my
occupational interest has been in
developing the hotel industry which
was the source of success in my life
until 2005.  Four years prior to being
diagnosed with Parkinson's disease in
2003, I had a strong suspicion that I
might be developing symptoms of
Parkinson's.  You see, my father had
Parkinson's so I had a firsthand
knowledge about symptoms he
experienced that I too now was
beginning to experience.*

*My business and expertise was in the*

*hotel business. Looking into future business needs, I encouraged my son to seek a rewarding and fruitful business that dictated the future needs of many baby-boomers. With my help, my son has become successful in building 3 phases of a retirement home with plans to expand into another nearby city. I am quite involved with the maintenance of the building and overseeing many of the building projects that has grown with our family. It is wonderful and I am blessed to be involved in the care and lives of my two grandsons as they learn the business first hand from family. Connecting with the seniors enhances my day. Those with Parkinson's have given me a common bond to understand and communicate with those in common.*

*Keeping fit has always been important to me. I started my spare time courier martial arts and enjoy today a 4.3 degree black belt credential and am working to achieve a 4.4 credential by November, 2011. I have enjoyed being a martial arts instructor since 1998. I felt it was important to prepare myself and out of defiance started scuba diving in 2006. In 2008 I was awarded the title of master diver.*

*My stubbornness and defiance of this disease gave me the courage to coach my grandson in martial arts. I am very proud that he achieved his black belt in 2010 at 12 years of age. As is evident from the interview, my persistent and determined personality is part of managing this disease. You can contact me through my email address: info@gesumo.com*

www.ingramcontent.com/pod-product-compliance
Lightning Source LLC
Chambersburg PA
CBHW070342290526
45791CB00003B/1444